The Plant Based Diet Recipe Book For Advanced

Best Delicious Plant-Based Diet Recipe Book for Advanced Users. Eat Healthier, Get Fit and Lose Weight Fast

Valerie Harvey

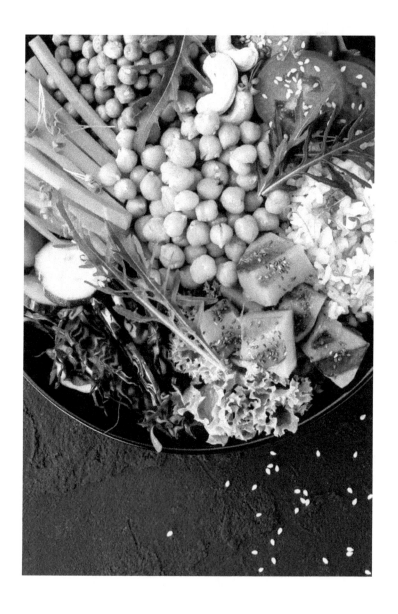

Table of Contents

The information in the following pages is broadly considered a truthful and accurate account of facts and as such, any inattention, use, or misuse of the information in question by the reader will render any resulting actions solely under their purview. There are no scenarios in which the publisher or the original author of this work can be in any fashion deemed liable for any hardship or damages that may befall them after undertaking information described herein.

Additionally, the information in the following pages is intended only for informational purposes and should thus be thought of as universal. As befitting its nature, it is presented without assurance regarding its prolonged validity or interim quality. Trademarks that are mentioned are done without written consent and can in no way be considered an endorsement from the trademark holder.

Introduction

A plant-based diet is a diet based primarily on whole plant foods. It is identical to the regular diet we're used to already, except that it leaves out foods that are not exclusively from plants. Hence, a plant-based diet does away with all types of animal-sourced foods, hydrogenated oils, refined sugars, and processed foods. A whole food plant-based diet comprises not just fruits and vegetables; it also consists of unprocessed or barely-processed oils with healthy monounsaturated fats (like extra-virgin olive oil), whole grains, legumes (essentially lentils and beans), seeds and nuts, as well as herbs and spices.

What makes a plant-based meal (or any meal) fun is the manner with which you make them; the seasoning process; and the combination process that contributes to a fantastic flavor and makes every meal unique and enjoyable. There are lots of delicious recipes (all plant-centered), which will prove helpful in when you intend making mouthwatering, healthy plant-based dishes for personal or household consumption. Provided you're eating these plant-based foods regularly, you'll have very problems with fat or diseases that result from bad dietary habits, and there would be no need for excessive calorie tracking.

Plant-based diet recipes are versatile; they range from colorful Salads to Lentil Stews, and Bean Burritos. The recipes also draw influences from around the globe, with Mexican, Chinese, European, Indian cuisines all part of the vast array of plant-based recipes available to choose from. Why You Ought to Reduce Your Intake of Processed and Animal-Based Foods. You have likely heard over and over that processed food has adverse effects on your health. You might have also been told repeatedly to stay away from foods with lots of preservatives; nevertheless, nobody ever offered any genuine or concrete facts about why you ought to avoid these foods and why they are unsafe. Consequently, let us properly dissect it to help you properly comprehend why you ought to stay away from these healthy eating offenders. They have massive habit-forming characteristics. Humans have a predisposition towards being addicted to some specific foods; however, the reality is that the fault is not wholly ours. Every one of the unhealthy treats we relish now and then triggers the dopamine release in our brains. This creates a pleasurable effect in our brain, but the excitement is usually short-lived. The discharged dopamine additionally causes an attachment connection gradually, and this is the reason some people consistently go back to eat certain unhealthy foods even when they know it's unhealthy and unnecessary.

You can get rid of this by taking out that inducement completely. They are sugar-laden and plenteous in glucose-fructose syrup. Animal-based and processed foods are laden with refined sugars and glucose-fructose syrup which has almost no beneficial food nutrient. An ever-increasing number of studies are affirming what several people presumed from the start; that genetically modified foods bring about inflammatory bowel disease, which consequently makes it increasingly difficult for the body to assimilate essential nutrients. The disadvantages that result from your body being unable to assimilate essential nutrients from consumed foods rightly cannot be overemphasized. Processed and animal-based food products contain plenteous amounts of refined carbohydrates. Indeed, your body requires carbohydrates to give it the needed energy to run body capacities. In any case, refining carbs dispenses with the fundamental supplements; in the way that refining entire grains disposes of the whole grain part. What remains, in the wake of refining, is what's considered as empty carbs or empty calories. These can negatively affect the metabolic system in your body by sharply increasing your blood sugar and insulin quantities. They contain lots of synthetic ingredients. At the point when your body is taking in non-natural ingredients, it regards them as foreign substances.

Your body treats them as a health threat. Your body isn't accustomed to identifying synthetic compounds like sucralose or these synthesized sugars. Hence, in defense of your health against this foreign "aggressor," your body does what it's capable of to safeguard your health. It sets off an immune reaction to tackle this "enemy" compound, which indirectly weakens your body's general disease alertness, making you susceptible to illnesses. The concentration and energy expended by your body in ensuring your immune system remain safe could instead be devoted somewhere else. They contain constituent elements that set off an excitable reward sensation in your body. A part of processed and animal-based foods contain compounds like glucose-fructose syrup, monosodium glutamate, and specific food dyes that can trigger some addiction. They rouse your body to receive a benefit in return whenever you consume them. Monosodium glutamate, for example, is added to many store-bought baked foods. This additive slowly conditions your palates to relish the taste. It gets mental just by how your brain interrelates with your taste sensors.

This reward-centric arrangement makes you crave it increasingly, which ends up exposing you to the danger of over consuming calories.

For animal protein, usually, the expression "subpar" is used to allude to plant proteins since they generally have lower levels of essential amino acids as against animal-sourced protein. Nevertheless, what the vast majority don't know is that large amounts of essential amino acids can prove detrimental to your health. Let me break it down further for you.

Three-Bean Chili

Preparation Time: 5 Minutes

Cooking Time: 55 Minutes

Serving: 4

Ingredients:

   1 tablespoon extra-virgin olive oil

   1 medium yellow onion, chopped

   3 garlic cloves, minced

   1 (28-ounce) can crushed tomatoes

   1 (4-ounce) can chopped mild green chiles, drained

   1 cup water

   3 tablespoons chili powder

   1 canned chipotle chile in adobo, minced

   1 teaspoon ground cumin

   1/2 teaspoon dried marjoram

   1 1/2 cups cooked or 1 (15.5-ounce) can black beans,
      drained and rinsed

   1 1/2 cups cooked or 1 (15.5-ounce) can Great Northern
      or other white beans, drained and rinsed

   1 1/2 cups cooked or 1 (15.5-ounce) can dark red
      kidney beans, drained and rinsed

   Salt and freshly ground black pepper

Directions:

In a large saucepan, heat the oil over medium heat. Add the onion and garlic, cover, and cook until softened, about 7 minutes.

Add the tomatoes, green chiles, water, chili powder, chipotle, cumin, marjoram, and sugar.

Stir in the black beans, Great Northern beans, and kidney beans, then season with salt and pepper.

Bring to boil, then reduce the heat to low and simmer, uncovered while stirring occasionally for 45 minutes.

Uncover, and cook an additional 10 minutes to allow flavors to develop and for the chili to thicken. Serve immediately.

Nutrition:

Calories: 260

Total Fat: 14g

Carbs: 30g

Fiber: 10g

Protein: 12g

Chinese Black Bean Chili

Preparation Time: 15 Minutes

Cooking Time: 0 Minutes

Serving: 4

Ingredients:

1 tablespoon extra-virgin olive oil

1 medium yellow onion, finely chopped

2 medium carrots, finely chopped

1 teaspoon grated fresh ginger

2 tablespoons chili powder

1 teaspoon brown sugar

1 (28-ounce) can diced tomatoes, undrained

1/2 cup Chinese black bean sauce

3/4 cup water

4 1/2 cups cooked or 3 (15.5-ounce) cans black beans, drained and rinsed

Salt and freshly ground black pepper

2 tablespoons minced green onion, for garnish

Directions:

In a large pot, heat the oil over medium heat. Add the onion and carrot. Cover and cook until softened for about 10 minutes.

Stir in the ginger, chili powder, and sugar. Add the
tomatoes, black bean sauce, and water. Stir in the
black beans and season with salt and pepper.

Bring to boil, then reduce the heat to medium and
simmer, covered, until the vegetables are tender for
about 30 minutes.

Simmer for about 10 minutes longer. Serve
immediately garnished with green onion.

Nutrition:

Calories: 360

Total Fat: 13g

Carbs: 40g

Fiber: 9g

Protein: 14g

New World Chili

Preparation Time: 5 Minutes

Cooking Time: 55 Minutes

Serving: 4

Ingredients:

   1 small butternut squash, peeled, halved, and seeded

   1 tablespoon extra-virgin olive oil

   1 medium onion, chopped

   3 cups mild tomato salsa, homemade or store-bought

   3 cups cooked or 2 (15.5-ounce) cans pinto beans,
      drained and rinsed

   1 cup frozen lima beans

   1 cup fresh or frozen corn kernels

   1 canned chipotle chile in adobo, minced

   1 cup water

   3 tablespoons chili powder

   1/2 teaspoon ground allspice

   1/2 teaspoon sugar

   Salt and freshly ground black pepper

Directions:

   Cut the squash into 1/4-inch dice and set aside. In a
      large saucepan, heat the oil over medium heat.

   Add the onion and squash, cover, then cook until
      softened for about 10 minutes.

Add the salsa, pinto beans, lima beans, corn, and
chipotle chile. Stir chili powder, allspice, sugar, and
salt and black pepper into the water.

Bring to boil, then reduce the heat to medium and
simmer, covered, until the vegetables are tender for
about 45 minutes.

Uncover and simmer for about 10 minutes longer.
Serve immediately.

Nutrition:

Calories: 298

Total Fat: 19g

Carbs: 30g

Fiber: 10g

Protein: 15g

Lentil Salad With Chiles

Preparation Time: 5 Minutes

Cooking Time: 40 Minutes

Serving: 4

Ingredients:

   1 cup brown lentils, picked over, rinsed, and drained

   4 ripe plum tomatoes, chopped

   2 celery ribs, cut into ¼-inch slices

   1 or 2 hot or mild chiles, seeded and minced

   1/3 cup chopped green onions

   2 tablespoons chopped fresh parsley

   4 tablespoons olive oil

   2 tablespoons sherry or balsamic vinegar

   Salt and freshly ground black pepper

Directions:

   Bring a medium saucepan of salted water to boil over high heat. Add the lentils, return to a boil, then reduce to low.

   Cover and cook until the lentils are tender for about 40 minutes.

   Drain the lentils well and transfer to a large bowl. Add the tomatoes, celery, chiles, green onions, parsley, oil, and vinegar.

Season with salt and pepper, then toss well to combine
and serve

Nutrition:

Calories: 380

Total Fat: 12g

Carbs: 20g

Fiber: 11g

Protein: 15g

Black Bean And Corn Salad With Cilantro Dressing

Preparation Time: 15 Minutes

Cooking Time: 0 Minutes

Serving: 4

Ingredients:

2 cups frozen corn, thawed

3 cups cooked or 2 (15.5-ounce) cans black beans, rinsed and drained

1/2 cup chopped red bell pepper

1/4 cup minced red onion

1 (4-ounce) can chopped mild green chiles, drained

2 garlic cloves, crushed

1/4 cup chopped fresh cilantro

1 teaspoon ground cumin

1/2 teaspoon salt (optional)

1/4 teaspoon freshly ground black pepper

2 tablespoons fresh lime juice

2 tablespoons water

1/4 cup extra-virgin olive oil

Directions:

In a large bowl, combine the corn, beans, bell pepper, onion, and chiles. Set aside.

In a blender or food processor, mince the garlic. Add the cilantro, cumin, salt, and black pepper, then pulse to blend.

Add the lime juice, water, and oil and process until well blended.

Pour the dressing over the salad and toss to combine. Taste and adjust the seasonings if necessary, then serve.

Nutrition:

Calories: 260

Total Fat: 14g

Carbs: 38g

Fiber: 12g

Protein: 15g

Jerk-Spiced Red Bean Chili

Preparation Time: 5 Minutes

Cooking Time: 50 Minutes

Serving: 4

Ingredients:

   1 tablespoon extra-virgin olive oil

   1 medium onion, chopped

   8 ounces seitan, chopped

   3 cups cooked or 2 (15.5-ounce) cans dark red kidney
      beans, drained and rinsed

   1 (14.5-ounce) can crushed tomatoes

   1 (14.5-ounce) can diced tomatoes, drained

   1 (4-ounce) can chopped mild or hot green chiles,
      drained

   1/2 cup barbecue sauce

   1 cup water

   1 tablespoon soy sauce

   1 tablespoon chili powder

   1 teaspoon ground cumin

   1 teaspoon ground allspice

   1/2 teaspoon ground oregano

   1/4 teaspoon ground cayenne

   1/2 teaspoon salt

   1/4 teaspoon freshly ground black pepper

Directions:

In a large pot, heat the oil over medium heat. Add the onion and seitan.

Cover and cook until the onion is softened for about 10 minutes.

Stir in the kidney beans, crushed tomatoes, diced tomatoes, and chiles.

Stir in the barbecue sauce, water, soy sauce, chili powder, cumin, allspice, sugar, oregano, cayenne, salt, and black pepper.

Bring to boil, then reduce the heat to medium and simmer, covered, until the vegetables are tender for about 45 minutes.

Uncover and simmer about 10 minutes longer. Serve immediately.

Nutrition:

Calories: 340

Total Fat: 19g

Carbs: 70g

Fiber: 10g

Protein: 15g

Warm Lentil Salad With Walnuts

Preparation Time: 5 Minutes

Cooking Time: 45 Minutes

Serving: 4

Ingredients:

    1 cup green lentils, picked over, rinsed, and drained

    1 medium shallot, halved

    1 garlic clove, crushed

    2 tablespoons white wine vinegar

    1 tablespoon Dijon mustard

    1/4 cup extra-virgin olive oil

    1/2 teaspoon dried oregano

    1/2 teaspoon salt

    1/4 teaspoon freshly ground black pepper

    1/2 cup finely chopped red bell pepper

    1/3 cup chopped toasted walnuts

    1/4 cup finely chopped red onion

    2 tablespoons minced fresh parsley

Directions:

Bring a medium saucepan of salted water to boil. Add the lentils and return to boil, then reduce the heat to low.

Cover and cook until lentils are tender for about 45 minutes.

In a blender or food processor, mince the shallot and
garlic.

Add the vinegar, mustard, oil, oregano, salt, and black
pepper, then process until well blended. Set aside.

When the lentils are tender, drain well and transfer to
a serving bowl. Add the bell pepper, walnuts,
onion, and parsley.

Nutrition:

Calories: 360

Total Fat: 13g

Carbs: 20g

Fiber: 12g

Protein: 14g

Lemon and Thyme Couscous

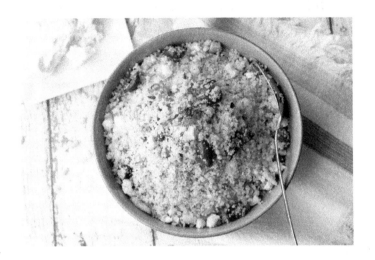

Preparation Time: 5 Minutes

Cooking Time: 10 Minutes

Serving: 6

Ingredients:

   2 3/4 cups vegetable stock

   Juice and zest of 1 lemon

   2 tablespoons chopped fresh thyme

   1 1/2 cups couscous

   1/4 cup chopped fresh parsley

   Sea salt

   Freshly ground black pepper

Directions:

In a medium pot, bring the vegetable stock, lemon
juice, and thyme to a boil. Stir in the couscous,
cover, and remove from the heat.

Allow to sit, covered, until the -couscous absorbs the
liquid and softens, about 5 minutes. Fluff with a
fork.

Stir in the lemon zest and parsley. Season with salt and
pepper. Serve hot.

Nutrition:

Calories: 290

Total Fat: 19g

Carbs: 10g

Fiber: 10g

Protein: 15g

Legumes

Traditional Indian Rajma Dal

Preparation Time: 5 Minutes
Cooking Time: 20 Minutes
Serving: 4
Ingredients:

   3 tablespoons sesame oil

   1 teaspoon ginger, minced

   1 teaspoon cumin seeds

   1 teaspoon coriander seeds

   1 large onion, chopped

   1 celery stalk, chopped

   1 teaspoon garlic, minced

   1 cup tomato sauce

   1 teaspoon garam masala

   1/2 teaspoon curry powder

   1 small cinnamon stick

   1 green chili, seeded and minced

   2 cups canned red kidney beans, drained

   2 cups vegetable broth

   Kosher salt and ground black pepper, to taste

Directions:

In a saucepan, heat the sesame oil over medium-high
heat; now, sauté the ginger, cumin seeds and
coriander seeds until fragrant or about 30 seconds
or so.

Add in the onion and celery and continue to sauté for 3
minutes more until they've softened.

Add in the garlic and continue to sauté for 1 minute
longer.

Stir the remaining **Ingredients:** into the saucepan
and turn the heat to a simmer. Continue to cook for
10 to 12 minutes or until thoroughly cooked. Serve
warm and enjoy!

Nutrition:

Calories: 269

Fat: 15.2g

Carbs: 22.9g

Protein: 7.2g

Red Kidney Bean Salad

Preparation Time: 20 Minutes

Cooking Time: 1 hour

Serving: 6

Ingredients:

3/4 pound red kidney beans, soaked overnight

2 bell peppers, chopped

1 carrot, trimmed and grated

3 ounces frozen or canned corn kernels, drained

3 heaping tablespoons scallions, chopped

2 cloves garlic, minced

1 red chile pepper, sliced

1/2 cup extra-virgin olive oil

2 tablespoons apple cider vinegar

2 tablespoons fresh lemon juice

Sea salt and ground black pepper, to taste

2 tablespoons fresh cilantro, chopped

2 tablespoons fresh parsley, chopped

2 tablespoons fresh basil, chopped

Directions:

Cover the soaked beans with a fresh change of cold water and bring to a boil. Let it boil for about 10 minutes.

Turn the heat to a simmer and continue to cook for 50 to 55 minutes or until tender.

Allow your beans to cool completely, then, transfer them to a salad bowl.

Add in the remaining **Ingredients:** and toss to combine well. Bon appétit!

Nutrition:

Calories: 443

Fat: 19.2g

Carbs: 52.2g

Protein: 18.1g

Anasazi Bean and Vegetable Stew

Preparation Time: 10 Minutes

Cooking Time: 1 hour

Serving: 4

Ingredients:

- 1 cup Anasazi beans, soaked overnight and drained
- 3 cups roasted vegetable broth
- 1 bay laurel
- 1 thyme sprig, chopped
- 1 rosemary sprig, chopped
- 3 tablespoons olive oil
- 1 large onion, chopped
- 2 celery stalks, chopped
- 2 carrots, chopped
- 2 bell peppers, seeded and chopped
- 1 green chili pepper, seeded and chopped
- 2 garlic cloves, minced
- Sea salt and ground black pepper, to taste
- 1 teaspoon cayenne pepper
- 1 teaspoon paprika

Directions:

In a saucepan, bring the Anasazi beans and broth to a boil. Once boiling, turn the heat to a simmer.

Add in the bay laurel, thyme and rosemary; let it cook for about 50 minutes or until tender.

Meanwhile, in a heavy-bottomed pot, heat the olive oil over medium-high heat.

Now, sauté the onion, celery, carrots and peppers for about 4 minutes until tender.

Add in the garlic and continue to sauté for 30 seconds more or until aromatic.

Add the sautéed mixture to the cooked beans. Season with salt, black pepper, cayenne pepper and paprika.

Continue to simmer, stirring periodically, for 10 minutes more or until everything is cooked through.

Nutrition:

Calories: 444

Fat: 15.8g

Carbs: 58.2g

Protein: 20.2g

Easy and Hearty Shakshuka

Preparation Time: 10 Minutes

Cooking Time: 50 Minutes

Serving: 4

Ingredients:

   2 tablespoons olive oil

   1 onion, chopped

   2 bell peppers, chopped

   1 poblano pepper, chopped

   2 cloves garlic, minced

   2 tomatoes, pureed

   Sea salt and black pepper, to taste

   1 teaspoon dried basil

   1 teaspoon red pepper flakes

   1 teaspoon paprika

   2 bay leaves

   1 cup chickpeas, soaked overnight, rinsed and drained

   3 cups vegetable broth

   2 tablespoons fresh cilantro, roughly chopped

Directions:

Heat the olive oil in a saucepan over medium heat.
   Once hot, cook the onion, peppers and garlic for
   about 4 minutes, until tender and aromatic.

Add in the pureed tomato tomatoes, sea salt, black
pepper, basil, red pepper, paprika and bay leaves.

Turn the heat to a simmer and add in the chickpeas
and vegetable broth. Cook for 45 minutes or until
tender.

Taste and adjust seasonings. Spoon your shakshuka
into individual bowls and serve garnished with the
fresh cilantro.

Nutrition:

Calories: 324

Fat: 11.2g

Carbs: 42.2g

Protein: 15.8g

Old-Fashioned Chili

Preparation Time: 15 Minutes

Cooking Time: 1 hour 30 Minutes

Serving: 6

Ingredients:

3/4 pound red kidney beans, soaked overnight

2 tablespoons olive oil

1 onion, chopped

2 bell peppers, chopped

1 red chili pepper, chopped

2 ribs celery, chopped

2 cloves garlic, minced

2 bay leaves

1 teaspoon ground cumin

1 teaspoon thyme, chopped

1 teaspoon black peppercorns

20 ounces tomatoes, crushed

2 cups vegetable broth

1 teaspoon smoked paprika

Sea salt, to taste

2 tablespoons fresh cilantro, chopped

1 avocado, pitted, peeled and sliced

Directions:

Cover the soaked beans with a fresh change of cold water and bring to a boil. Let it boil for about 10 minutes.

Turn the heat to a simmer and continue to cook for 50 to 55 minutes or until tender.

In a heavy-bottomed pot, heat the olive oil over medium heat. Once hot, sauté the onion, bell pepper and celery.

Sauté the garlic, bay leaves, ground cumin, thyme and black peppercorns for about 1 minute or so.

Add in the diced tomatoes, vegetable broth, paprika, salt and cooked beans.

Let it simmer, stirring periodically, for 25 to 30 minutes or until cooked through.

Serve garnished with fresh cilantro and avocado.

Nutrition:

Calories: 514

Fat: 16.4g

Carbs: 72g

Protein: 25.8g

Easy Red Lentil Salad

Preparation Time: 5 Minutes

Cooking Time: 20 Minutes

Serving: 3

Ingredients:

1/2 cup red lentils, soaked overnight and drained

1 1/2 cups water

1 sprig rosemary

1 bay leaf

1 cup grape tomatoes, halved

1 cucumber, thinly sliced

1 bell pepper, thinly sliced

1 clove garlic, minced

1 onion, thinly sliced

2 tablespoons fresh lime juice

4 tablespoons olive oil

Sea salt and ground black pepper, to taste

Directions:

Add the red lentils, water, rosemary and bay leaf to a saucepan and bring to a boil over high heat.

Then, turn the heat to a simmer and continue to cook for 20 minutes or until tender.

Place the lentils in a salad bowl and let them cool completely.

Add in the remaining **Ingredients:** and toss to combine well. Serve at room temperature or well-chilled.

Nutrition:

Calories: 295

Fat: 18.8g

Carbs: 25.2g

Protein: 8.5g

Mediterranean-Style Chickpea Salad

Preparation Time: 5 Minutes

Cooking Time: 40 Minutes

Serving: 4

Ingredients:

   2 cups chickpeas, soaked overnight and drained

   1 Persian cucumber, sliced

   1 cup cherry tomatoes, halved

   1 red bell peppers, seeded and sliced

   1 green bell pepper, seeded and sliced

   1 teaspoon deli mustard

   1 teaspoon coriander seeds

   1 teaspoon jalapeno pepper, minced

   1 tablespoon fresh lemon juice

   1 tablespoon balsamic vinegar

   1/4 cup extra-virgin olive oil

   Sea salt and ground black pepper, to taste

   2 tablespoons fresh cilantro, chopped

   2 tablespoons Kalamata olives, pitted and sliced

Directions:

Place the chickpeas in a stockpot; cover the chickpeas
   with water by 2 inches. Bring it to a boil.

Immediately turn the heat to a simmer and continue to
   cook for about 40 minutes or until tender.

Transfer your chickpeas to a salad bowl. Add in the remaining **Ingredients:** and toss to combine well.

Nutrition:

Calories: 468

Fat: 12.5g

Carbs: 73g

Protein: 21.8g

Traditional Tuscan Bean Stew (Ribollita)

Preparation Time: 5 Minutes
Cooking Time: 25 Minutes
Serving: 5
Ingredients:

> 3 tablespoons olive oil
>
> 1 medium leek, chopped
>
> 1 celery with leaves, chopped
>
> 1 zucchini, diced
>
> 1 Italian pepper, sliced
>
> 3 garlic cloves, crushed
>
> 2 bay leaves
>
> Kosher salt and ground black pepper, to taste
>
> 1 teaspoon cayenne pepper
>
> 1 (28-ounce) can tomatoes, crushed
>
> 2 cups vegetable broth
>
> 2 (15-ounce) cans Great Northern beans, drained
>
> 2 cups Lacinato kale, torn into pieces
>
> 1 cup crostini

Directions:

> In a heavy-bottomed pot, heat the olive oil over medium heat. Once hot, sauté the leek, celery, zucchini and pepper for about 4 minutes.

Sauté the garlic and bay leaves for about 1 minute or
so.

Add in the spices, tomatoes, broth and canned beans.
Let it simmer, stirring occasionally, for about 15
minutes or until cooked through.

Add in the Lacinato kale and continue simmering,
stirring occasionally, for 4 minutes.

Serve garnished with crostini.

Nutrition:

Calories: 388

Fat: 10.3g

Carbs: 57.3g

Protein: 19.5g

Beluga Lentil and Vegetable Mélange

Preparation Time: 10 Minutes

Cooking Time: 25 Minutes

Serving: 5

Ingredients:

    3 tablespoons olive oil

    1 onion, minced

    2 bell peppers, seeded and chopped

    1 carrot, trimmed and chopped

    1 parsnip, trimmed and chopped

    1 teaspoon ginger, minced

    2 cloves garlic, minced

    Sea salt and ground black pepper, to taste

    1 large-sized zucchini, diced

    1 cup tomato sauce

    1 cup vegetable broth

    1 1/2 cups beluga lentils, soaked overnight and drained

    2 cups Swiss chard

Directions:

    In a Dutch oven, heat the olive oil until sizzling. Now,
        sauté the onion, bell pepper, carrot and parsnip,
        until they've softened.

    Add in the ginger and garlic and continue sautéing an
        additional 30 seconds.

Now, add in the salt, black pepper, zucchini, tomato sauce, vegetable broth and lentils; let it simmer for about 20 minutes until everything is thoroughly cooked.

Add in the Swiss chard; cover and let it simmer for 5 minutes more.

Nutrition:

Calories: 382

Fat: 9.3g

Carbs: 59g

Protein: 17.2g

Mexican Chickpea Taco Bowls

Preparation Time: 5 Minutes

Cooking Time: 15 Minutes

Serving: 4

Ingredients:

2 tablespoons sesame oil

1 red onion, chopped

1 habanero pepper, minced

2 garlic cloves, crushed

2 bell peppers, seeded and diced

Sea salt and ground black pepper

1/2 teaspoon Mexican oregano

1 teaspoon ground cumin

2 ripe tomatoes, pureed

1 teaspoon brown sugar

16 ounces canned chickpeas, drained

4 (8-inch) flour tortillas

2 tablespoons fresh coriander, roughly chopped

Directions:

In a large skillet, heat the sesame oil over a moderately high heat. Then, sauté the onions for 2 to 3 minutes or until tender.

Add in the peppers and garlic and continue to sauté for 1 minute or until fragrant.

Add in the spices, tomatoes and brown sugar and bring to a boil.

Immediately turn the heat to a simmer, add in the canned chickpeas and let it cook for 8 minutes longer or until heated through.

Toast your tortillas and arrange them with the prepared chickpea mixture.

Top with fresh coriander and serve immediately.

Nutrition:

Calories: 409

Fat: 13.5g

Carbs: 61.3g

Protein: 13.8g

Indian Dal Makhani

Preparation Time: 10 minutes

Cooking Time: 10 minutes

Servings: 4

Ingredients:

- 3 tablespoons sesame oil
- 1 large onion, chopped
- 1 bell pepper, seeded and chopped
- 2 garlic cloves, minced
- 1 tablespoon ginger, grated
- 2 green chilies, seeded and chopped
- 1 teaspoon cumin seeds
- 1 bay laurel
- 1 teaspoon turmeric powder
- 1/4 teaspoon red peppers
- 1/4 teaspoon ground allspice
- 1/2 teaspoon garam masala
- 1 cup tomato sauce
- 4 cups vegetable broth
- 1 ½ cups black lentils, soaked overnight and drained
- 4-5 curry leaves, for garnish

Directions

1. In a saucepan, heat the sesame oil over medium-high heat; now, sauté the onion and bell pepper for 3 minutes more until they've softened.

2. Add in the garlic, ginger, green chilies, cumin seeds and bay laurel; continue to sauté, stirring frequently, for 1 minute or until fragrant.

3. Stir in the remaining ingredients, except for the curry leaves. Now, turn the heat to a simmer. Continue to cook for 15 minutes more or until thoroughly cooked.

4. Garnish with curry leaves and serve hot!

Nutrition:

Calories: 329; Fat: 8.5g; Carbs: 44.1g; Protein: 16.8g

Mexican-Style Bean Bowl

Preparation Time: 10 minutes

Cooking Time: 10 minutes

Servings: 4

Ingredients:

- 1 pound red beans, soaked overnight and drained
- 1 cup canned corn kernels, drained
- 2 roasted bell peppers, sliced
- 1 chili pepper, finely chopped
- 1 cup cherry tomatoes, halved
- 1 red onion, chopped
- 1/4 cup fresh cilantro, chopped
- 1/4 cup fresh parsley, chopped
- 1 teaspoon Mexican oregano
- 1/4 cup red wine vinegar
- 2 tablespoons fresh lemon juice
- 1/3 cup extra-virgin olive oil
- Sea salt and ground black, to taste
- 1 avocado, peeled, pitted and sliced

Directions

1. Cover the soaked beans with a fresh change of cold water and bring to a boil. Let it boil for about 10 minutes. Turn the heat to a simmer and continue to cook for 50 to 55 minutes or until tender.

2. Allow your beans to cool completely, then, transfer them to a salad bowl.
3. Add in the remaining ingredients and toss to combine well. Serve at room temperature.
4. Bon appétit!

Nutrition:

Calories: 465; Fat: 17.9g; Carbs: 60.4g; Protein: 20.2g

Classic Italian Minestrone

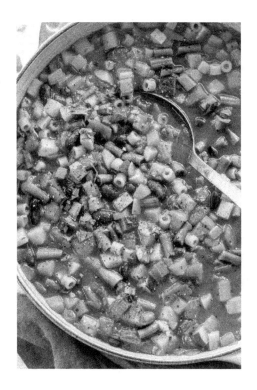

Preparation Time: 10 minutes

Cooking Time: 10 minutes

Servings: 4

Ingredients:

- 2 tablespoons olive oil
- 1 large onion, diced
- 2 carrots, sliced
- 4 cloves garlic, minced
- 1 cup elbow pasta

- 5 cups vegetable broth
- 1 (15-ounce) can white beans, drained
- 1 large zucchini, diced
- 1 (28-ounce) can tomatoes, crushed
- 1 tablespoon fresh oregano leaves, chopped
- 1 tablespoon fresh basil leaves, chopped
- 1 tablespoon fresh Italian parsley, chopped

Directions

1. In a Dutch oven, heat the olive oil until sizzling. Now, sauté the onion and carrots until they've softened.
2. Add in the garlic, uncooked pasta and broth; let it simmer for about 15 minutes.
3. Stir in the beans, zucchini, tomatoes and herbs. Continue to cook, covered, for about 10 minutes until everything is thoroughly cooked.
4. Garnish with some extra herbs, if desired. Bon appétit!

Nutrition:

Calories: 305; Fat: 8.6g; Carbs: 45.1g; Protein: 14.2g

Green Lentil Stew with Collard Greens

Preparation Time: 10 minutes

Cooking Time: 10 minutes

Servings: 4

Ingredients:

- 2 tablespoons olive oil
- 1 onion, chopped
- 2 sweet potatoes, peeled and diced
- 1 bell pepper, chopped
- 2 carrots, chopped
- 1 parsnip, chopped
- 1 celery, chopped
- 2 cloves garlic
- 1 ½ cups green lentils
- 1 tablespoon Italian herb mix
- 1 cup tomato sauce
- 5 cups vegetable broth
- 1 cup frozen corn
- 1 cup collard greens, torn into pieces

Directions

1. In a Dutch oven, heat the olive oil until sizzling. Now, sauté the onion, sweet potatoes, bell pepper, carrots, parsnip and celery until they've softened.

2. Add in the garlic and continue sautéing an additional 30 seconds.
3. Now, add in the green lentils, Italian herb mix, tomato sauce and vegetable broth; let it simmer for about 20 minutes until everything is thoroughly cooked.
4. Add in the frozen corn and collard greens; cover and let it simmer for 5 minutes more. Bon appétit!

Nutrition:

Calories: 415; Fat: 6.6g; Carbs: 71g; Protein: 18.4g

Chickpea Garden Vegetable Medley

Preparation Time: 10 minutes

Cooking Time: 10 minutes

Servings: 4

Ingredients:

- 2 tablespoons olive oil
- 1 onion, finely chopped
- 1 bell pepper, chopped
- 1 fennel bulb, chopped
- 3 cloves garlic, minced
- 2 ripe tomatoes, pureed
- 2 tablespoons fresh parsley, roughly chopped
- 2 tablespoons fresh basil, roughly chopped
- 2 tablespoons fresh coriander, roughly chopped
- 2 cups vegetable broth
- 14 ounces canned chickpeas, drained
- Kosher salt and ground black pepper, to taste
- 1/2 teaspoon cayenne pepper
- 1 teaspoon paprika
- 1 avocado, peeled and sliced

Directions

1. In a heavy-bottomed pot, heat the olive oil over medium heat. Once hot, sauté the onion, bell pepper and fennel bulb for about 4 minutes.
2. Sauté the garlic for about 1 minute or until aromatic.

---

3. Add in the tomatoes, fresh herbs, broth, chickpeas, salt, black pepper, cayenne pepper and paprika. Let it simmer, stirring occasionally, for about 20 minutes or until cooked through.
4. Taste and adjust the seasonings. Serve garnished with the slices of the fresh avocado. Bon appétit!

Nutrition:

Calories: 369; Fat: 18.1g; Carbs: 43.5g; Protein: 13.2g

Hot Bean Dipping Sauce

Preparation Time: 10 minutes

Cooking Time: 10 minutes

Servings: 4

Ingredients:

- 2 (15-ounce) cans Great Northern beans, drained
- 2 tablespoons olive oil
- 2 tablespoons Sriracha sauce
- 2 tablespoons nutritional yeast
- 4 ounces' vegan cream cheese
- 1/2 teaspoon paprika
- 1/2 teaspoon cayenne pepper
- 1/2 teaspoon ground cumin
- Sea salt and ground black pepper, to taste
- 4 ounces' tortilla chips

Directions

1. Start by preheating your oven to 360 degrees F.
2. Pulse all the ingredients, except for the tortilla chips, in your food processor until your desired consistency is reached.
3. Bake your dip in the preheated oven for about 25 minutes or until hot.
4. Serve with tortilla chips and enjoy!

Nutrition: Calories: 175; Fat: 4.7g; Carbs: 24.9g; Protein: 8.8g

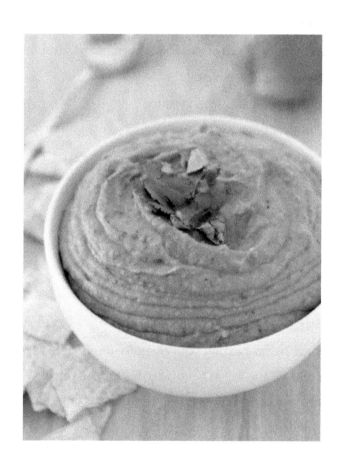

Chinese-Style Soybean Salad

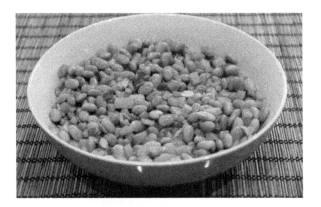

Preparation Time: 10 minutes

Cooking Time: 10 minutes

Servings: 4

Ingredients:

- 1 (15-ounce) can soybeans, drained
- 1 cup arugula
- 1 cup baby spinach
- 1 cup green cabbage, shredded
- 1 onion, thinly sliced
- 1/2 teaspoon garlic, minced
- 1 teaspoon ginger, minced
- 1/2 teaspoon deli mustard
- 2 tablespoons soy sauce
- 1 tablespoon rice vinegar
- 1 tablespoon lime juice

- 2 tablespoons tahini
- 1 teaspoon agave syrup

Directions

1. In a salad bowl, place the soybeans, arugula, spinach, cabbage and onion; toss to combine.
2. In a small mixing dish, whisk the remaining ingredients for the dressing.
3. Dress your salad and serve immediately. Bon appétit!

Nutrition: Calories: 265; Fat: 13.7g; Carbs: 21g; Protein: 18g

Old-Fashioned Lentil and Vegetable Stew

Preparation Time: 10 minutes

Cooking Time: 10 minutes

Servings: 4

Ingredients:

- 3 tablespoons olive oil
- 1 large onion, chopped
- 1 carrot, chopped
- 1 bell pepper, diced
- 1 habanero pepper, chopped
- 3 cloves garlic, minced
- Kosher salt and black pepper, to taste
- 1 teaspoon ground cumin
- 1 teaspoon smoked paprika
- 1 (28-ounce) can tomatoes, crushed
- 2 tablespoons tomato ketchup
- 4 cups vegetable broth
- 3/4 pound dry red lentils, soaked overnight and drained
- 1 avocado, sliced

Directions

1. In a heavy-bottomed pot, heat the olive oil over medium heat. Once hot, sauté the onion, carrot and peppers for about 4 minutes.
2. Sauté the garlic for about 1 minute or so.

3. Add in the spices, tomatoes, ketchup, broth and canned lentils. Let it simmer, stirring occasionally, for about 20 minutes or until cooked through.
4. Serve garnished with the slices of avocado. Bon appétit!

Nutrition: Calories: 475; Fat: 17.3g; Carbs: 61.4g; Protein: 23.7g

Indian Chana Masala

Preparation Time: 10 minutes

Cooking Time: 10 minutes

Servings: 4

Ingredients:

- 1 cup tomatoes, pureed
- 1 Kashmiri chile pepper, chopped
- 1 large shallot, chopped
- 1 teaspoon fresh ginger, peeled and grated
- 4 tablespoons olive oil
- 2 cloves garlic, minced
- 1 teaspoon coriander seeds
- 1 teaspoon garam masala
- 1/2 teaspoon turmeric powder
- Sea salt and ground black pepper, to taste
- 1/2 cup vegetable broth
- 16 ounces canned chickpeas
- 1 tablespoon fresh lime juice

Directions

1. In your blender or food processor, blend the tomatoes, Kashmiri chile pepper, shallot and ginger into a paste.
2. In a saucepan, heat the olive oil over medium heat. Once hot, cook the prepared paste and garlic for about 2 minutes.

3. Add in the remaining spices, broth and chickpeas. Turn the heat to a simmer. Continue to simmer for 8 minutes more or until cooked through.
4. Remove from the heat. Drizzle fresh lime juice over the top of each serving. Bon appétit!

Nutrition: Calories: 305; Fat: 17.1g; Carbs: 30.1g; Protein: 9.4g

Red Kidney Bean Pâté

Preparation Time: 10 minutes

Cooking Time: 10 minutes

Servings: 4

Ingredients:

- 2 tablespoons olive oil
- 1 onion, chopped
- 1 bell pepper, chopped
- 2 cloves garlic, minced
- 2 cups red kidney beans, boiled and drained
- 1/4 cup olive oil
- 1 teaspoon stone-ground mustard
- 2 tablespoons fresh parsley, chopped
- 2 tablespoons fresh basil, chopped
- Sea salt and ground black pepper, to taste

Directions

1. In a saucepan, heat the olive oil over medium-high heat. Now, cook the onion, pepper and garlic until just tender or about 3 minutes.
2. Add the sautéed mixture to your blender; add in the remaining ingredients. Puree the ingredients in your blender or food processor until smooth and creamy.
3. Bon appétit!

Nutrition: Calories: 135; Fat: 12.1g; Carbs: 4.4g; Protein: 1.6g

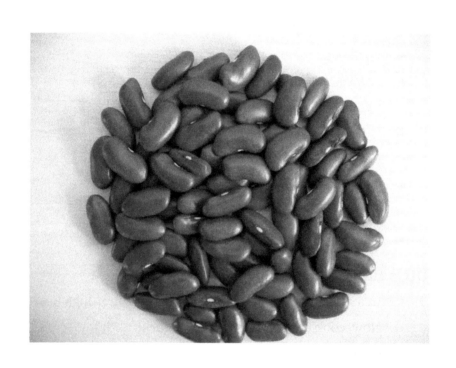

Brown Lentil Bowl

Preparation Time: 10 minutes

Cooking Time: 10 minutes

Servings: 4

Ingredients:

- 1 cup brown lentils, soaked overnight and drained
- 3 cups water
- 2 cups brown rice, cooked
- 1 zucchini, diced
- 1 red onion, chopped
- 1 teaspoon garlic, minced
- 1 cucumber, sliced
- 1 bell pepper, sliced
- 4 tablespoons olive oil
- 1 tablespoon rice vinegar
- 2 tablespoons lemon juice
- 2 tablespoons soy sauce
- 1/2 teaspoon dried oregano
- 1/2 teaspoon ground cumin
- Sea salt and ground black pepper, to taste
- 2 cups arugula
- 2 cups Romaine lettuce, torn into pieces

Directions

1. Add the brown lentils and water to a saucepan and bring to a boil over high heat. Then, turn the heat to a

simmer and continue to cook for 20 minutes or until tender.

2. Place the lentils in a salad bowl and let them cool completely.

3. Add in the remaining ingredients and toss to combine well. Serve at room temperature or well-chilled. Bon appétit!

Nutrition: Calories: 452; Fat: 16.6g; Carbs: 61.7g; Protein: 16.4g

Hot and Spicy Anasazi Bean Soup

Preparation Time: 10 minutes

Cooking Time: 10 minutes

Servings: 4

Ingredients:

- 2 cups Anasazi beans, soaked overnight, drained and rinsed
- 8 cups water
- 2 bay leaves
- 3 tablespoons olive oil
- 2 medium onions, chopped
- 2 bell peppers, chopped
- 1 habanero pepper, chopped
- 3 cloves garlic, pressed or minced
- Sea salt and ground black pepper, to taste

Directions

1. In a soup pot, bring the Anasazi beans and water to a boil. Once boiling, turn the heat to a simmer. Add in the bay leaves and let it cook for about 1 hour or until tender.
2. Meanwhile, in a heavy-bottomed pot, heat the olive oil over medium-high heat. Now, sauté the onion, peppers and garlic for about 4 minutes until tender.
3. Add the sautéed mixture to the cooked beans. Season with salt and black pepper.

4. Continue to simmer, stirring periodically, for 10 minutes more or until everything is cooked through. Bon appétit!

Nutrition: Calories: 352; Fat: 8.5g; Carbs: 50.1g; Protein: 19.7g

Black-Eyed Pea Salad (Ñebbe)

Preparation Time: 10 minutes

Cooking Time: 10 minutes

Servings: 4

Ingredients:

- 2 cups dried black-eyed peas, soaked overnight and drained
- 2 tablespoons basil leaves, chopped
- 2 tablespoons parsley leaves, chopped
- 1 shallot, chopped
- 1 cucumber, sliced
- 2 bell peppers, seeded and diced
- 1 Scotch bonnet chili pepper, seeded and finely chopped
- 1 cup cherry tomatoes, quartered
- Sea salt and ground black pepper, to taste
- 2 tablespoons fresh lime juice
- 1 tablespoon apple cider vinegar
- 1/4 cup extra-virgin olive oil
- 1 avocado, peeled, pitted and sliced

Directions

1. Cover the black-eyed peas with water by 2 inches and bring to a gentle boil. Let it boil for about 15 minutes.
2. Then, turn the heat to a simmer for about 45 minutes. Let it cool completely.

3. Place the black-eyed peas in a salad bowl. Add in the basil, parsley, shallot, cucumber, bell peppers, cherry tomatoes, salt and black pepper.
4. In a mixing bowl, whisk the lime juice, vinegar and olive oil.
5. Dress the salad, garnish with fresh avocado and serve immediately. Bon appétit!

Nutrition: Calories: 471; Fat: 17.5g; Carbs: 61.5g; Protein: 20.6g

Mom's Famous Chili

Preparation Time: 10 minutes

Cooking Time: 10 minutes

Servings: 4

Ingredients:

- 1 pound red black beans, soaked overnight and drained
- 3 tablespoons olive oil
- 1 large red onion, diced
- 2 bell peppers, diced
- 1 poblano pepper, minced
- 1 large carrot, trimmed and diced
- 2 cloves garlic, minced
- 2 bay leaves
- 1 teaspoon mixed peppercorns
- Kosher salt and cayenne pepper, to taste
- 1 tablespoon paprika
- 2 ripe tomatoes, pureed
- 2 tablespoons tomato ketchup
- 3 cups vegetable broth

Directions

1. Cover the soaked beans with a fresh change of cold water and bring to a boil. Let it boil for about 10 minutes. Turn the heat to a simmer and continue to cook for 50 to 55 minutes or until tender.

2. In a heavy-bottomed pot, heat the olive oil over medium heat. Once hot, sauté the onion, peppers and carrot.

3. Sauté the garlic for about 30 seconds or until aromatic.

4. Add in the remaining ingredients along with the cooked beans. Let it simmer, stirring periodically, for 25 to 30 minutes or until cooked through.

5. Discard the bay leaves, ladle into individual bowls and serve hot!

Nutrition: Calories: 455; Fat: 10.5g; Carbs: 68.6g; Protein: 24.7g

Creamed Chickpea Salad with Pine Nuts

Preparation Time: 10 minutes

Cooking Time: 10 minutes

Servings: 4

Ingredients:

- 16 ounces canned chickpeas, drained
- 1 teaspoon garlic, minced
- 1 shallot, chopped
- 1 cup cherry tomatoes, halved
- 1 bell pepper, seeded and sliced
- 1/4 cup fresh basil, chopped
- 1/4 cup fresh parsley, chopped
- 1/2 cup vegan mayonnaise
- 1 tablespoon lemon juice
- 1 teaspoon capers, drained
- Sea salt and ground black pepper, to taste
- 2 ounces' pine nuts

Directions

1. Place the chickpeas, vegetables and herbs in a salad bowl.
2. Add in the mayonnaise, lemon juice, capers, salt and black pepper. Stir to combine.
3. Top with pine nuts and serve immediately. Bon appétit!

Nutrition: Calories: 386; Fat: 22.5g; Carbs: 37.2g; Protein: 12.9g

Black Bean Buda Bowl

Preparation Time: 10 minutes

Cooking Time: 10 minutes

Servings: 4

Ingredients:

- 1/2 pound black beans, soaked overnight and drained
- 2 cups brown rice, cooked
- 1 medium-sized onion, thinly sliced
- 1 cup bell pepper, seeded and sliced
- 1 jalapeno pepper, seeded and sliced
- 2 cloves garlic, minced
- 1 cup arugula
- 1 cup baby spinach
- 1 teaspoon lime zest
- 1 tablespoon Dijon mustard
- 1/4 cup red wine vinegar
- 1/4 cup extra-virgin olive oil
- 2 tablespoons agave syrup
- Flaky sea salt and ground black pepper, to taste
- 1/4 cup fresh Italian parsley, roughly chopped

Directions

1. Cover the soaked beans with a fresh change of cold water and bring to a boil. Let it boil for about 10 minutes. Turn the heat to a simmer and continue to cook for 50 to 55 minutes or until tender.

2. To serve, divide the beans and rice between serving bowls; top with the vegetables.
3. A small mixing dish thoroughly combines the lime zest, mustard, vinegar, olive oil, agave syrup, salt and pepper. Drizzle the vinaigrette over the salad.
4. Garnish with fresh Italian parsley. Bon appétit!

Nutrition: Calories: 365; Fat: 14.1g; Carbs: 45.6g; Protein: 15.5g

Middle Eastern Chickpea Stew

Preparation Time: 10 minutes

Cooking Time: 10 minutes

Servings: 4

Ingredients:

- 1 onion, chopped
- 1 chili pepper, chopped
- 2 garlic cloves, chopped
- 1 teaspoon mustard seeds
- 1 teaspoon coriander seeds
- 1 bay leaf
- 1/2 cup tomato puree
- 2 tablespoons olive oil
- 1 celery with leaves, chopped
- 2 medium carrots, trimmed and chopped
- 2 cups vegetable broth
- 1 teaspoon ground cumin
- 1 small-sized cinnamon stick
- 16 ounces canned chickpeas, drained
- 2 cups Swiss chard, torn into pieces

Directions

1. In your blender or food processor, blend the onion, chili pepper, garlic, mustard seeds, coriander seeds, bay leaf and tomato puree into a paste.

2. In a stockpot, heat the olive oil until sizzling. Now, cook the celery and carrots for about 3 minutes or until they've softened. Add in the paste and continue to cook for a further 2 minutes.

3. Then, add vegetable broth, cumin, cinnamon and chickpeas; bring it to a gentle boil.

4. Turn the heat to simmer and let it cook for 6 minutes; fold in Swiss chard and continue to cook for 4 to 5 minutes more or until the leaves wilt. Serve hot and enjoy!

Nutrition: Calories: 305; Fat: 11.2g; Carbs: 38.6g; Protein: 12.7g

Lentil and Tomato Dip

Preparation Time: 10 minutes

Cooking Time: 10 minutes

Servings: 4

Ingredients:

- 16 ounces' lentils, boiled and drained
- 4 tablespoons sun-dried tomatoes, chopped
- 1 cup tomato paste
- 4 tablespoons tahini
- 1 teaspoon stone-ground mustard
- 1 teaspoon ground cumin
- 1/4 teaspoon ground bay leaf
- 1 teaspoon red pepper flakes
- Sea salt and ground black pepper, to taste

Directions

1. Blitz all the ingredients in your blender or food processor until your desired consistency is reached.
2. Place in your refrigerator until ready to serve.
3. Serve with toasted pita wedges or vegetable sticks. Enjoy!

Nutrition: Calories: 144; Fat: 4.5g; Carbs: 20.2g; Protein: 8.1g

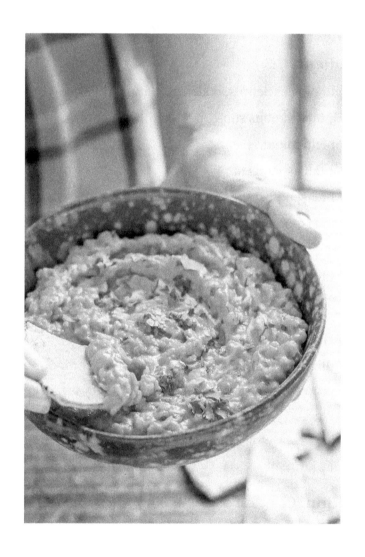

Creamed Green Pea Salad

Preparation Time: 10 minutes

Cooking Time: 10 minutes

Servings: 4

Ingredients:

- 2 (14.5 ounce) cans green peas, drained
- 1/2 cup vegan mayonnaise
- 1 teaspoon Dijon mustard
- 2 tablespoons scallions, chopped
- 2 pickles, chopped
- 1/2 cup marinated mushrooms, chopped and drained
- 1/2 teaspoon garlic, minced
- Sea salt and ground black pepper, to taste

Directions

1. Place all the ingredients in a salad bowl. Gently stir to combine.
2. Place the salad in your refrigerator until ready to serve.
3. Bon appétit!

Nutrition: Calories: 154; Fat: 6.7g; Carbs: 17.3g; Protein: 6.9g

Middle Eastern Za'atar Hummus

Preparation Time: 10 minutes

Cooking Time: 10 minutes

Servings: 4

Ingredients:

- 10 ounces' chickpeas, boiled and drained
- 1/4 cup tahini
- 2 tablespoons extra-virgin olive oil
- 2 tablespoons sun-dried tomatoes, chopped
- 1 lemon, freshly squeezed
- 2 garlic cloves, minced
- Kosher salt and ground black pepper, to taste
- 1/2 teaspoon smoked paprika
- 1 teaspoon Za'atar

Directions

Blitz all the ingredients in your food processor until creamy and uniform.

Place in your refrigerator until ready to serve.

Bon appétit!

Nutrition: Calories: 140; Fat: 8.5g; Carbs: 12.4g; Protein: 4.6g

Handhelds

Tofu Salad Sandwiches

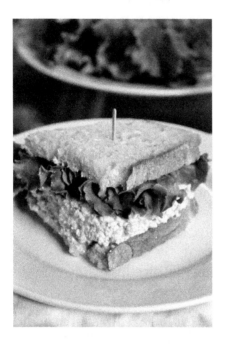

Preparation time: 15 minutes

Cooking time: 0 minutes

Servings: 6

Ingredients:

- 1 (14-ounce) package extra-firm tofu, drained and pressed (see here)

- 2 celery stalks, finely chopped

- 1 scallion, finely chopped

- 1/3 cup Cashew Mayonnaise, or store-bought nondairy mayonnaise

- 1 teaspoon yellow mustard

- 1 teaspoon freshly squeezed lemon juice

- 1 teaspoon ground turmeric

- Salt

- Freshly ground black pepper

- 12 slices bread of choice

- 1 large tomato, sliced

- 6 large romaine lettuce leaves

Directions:

1. Crumble the tofu into a medium bowl. Using a fork, gently mash it into small pieces.

2. Stir in the celery and scallion. Gently fold in the mayonnaise, mustard, lemon juice, and turmeric. Taste and season with salt and pepper.

3. Spoon the tofu mixture onto 6 slices of bread. Add the tomato slices and lettuce leaves and top with the remaining bread slices.

4. First-Timer tip: You can mix up your tofu salad by freezing the tofu beforehand, which makes it firmer and chewier. It also makes it a little spongy, which helps absorb dressings and sauces better. Just pop the package of tofu into the freezer. Once it's fully frozen, defrost it totally, then drain and press out the water as you normally would.

Nutrition:

Calories: 247;

Fat: 9g;

Carbohydrates: 30g;

Fiber: 5g;

Protein: 13g;

Sodium: 382mg;

Chickpea Salad Sandwiches

Preparation time: 15 minutes

Cooking time: 0 minutes

Servings: 4

Ingredients:

- 1 (15-ounce) can chickpeas, drained and rinsed, or 1½ cups cooked chickpeas (see here)

- 2 celery stalks, chopped

- 1 small carrot, grated or shredded

- 1/4 cup finely chopped red onion

- 1/4 cup finely chopped dill pickle, or pickle relish

- 1/4 cup Cashew Mayonnaise, or store-bought nondairy mayonnaise

- 1 teaspoon dried dill

- ½ teaspoon garlic powder

- ½ teaspoon onion powder

- Salt

- Freshly ground black pepper

- 8 slices bread of choice

- 1 large tomato, sliced

- 4 large romaine lettuce leaves

Directions:

1. Place the chickpeas in a large bowl and, using a potato masher or large fork, lightly mash them.

2. Gently stir in the celery, carrot, red onion, and dill pickle to combine everything.

3. Gently fold in the mayonnaise, dill, garlic powder, and onion powder. Taste and season with salt and pepper.

4. Spoon the chickpea mixture onto 4 slices of bread. Add the tomato slices and lettuce leaves and top with the remaining bread slices.

Nutrition:

Calories: 320;

Fat: 9g;

Carbohydrates: 49g;

Fiber: 10g;

Protein: 14g;

Sodium: 510mg;

Seitan Shawarma

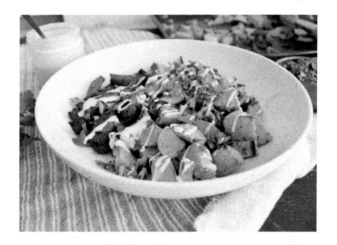

Preparation time: 20 minutes

Cooking time: 15 minutes

Servings: 4

Ingredients:

- 1/4 cup tahini

- 1/4 cup water

- 2 tablespoons freshly squeezed lemon juice

- 1 teaspoon garlic powder

- 2 teaspoons vegetable oil

- 1 small red onion, thinly sliced

- 1 pound Seitan, or store-bought seitan, thinly sliced

- 1/2 teaspoon ground cumin

- 1/2 teaspoon ground turmeric

- 1/2 teaspoon paprika

- 1/4 teaspoon salt

- ¼ teaspoon freshly ground black pepper

- 4 pitas, or flatbreads of choice

- 1 large tomato, sliced

- 1 cup sliced cucumber

- 2 cups sliced romaine lettuce

Directions:

1. In a small bowl, whisk the tahini, water, lemon juice, and garlic powder to blend. Set aside.

2. In a large pan over medium-high heat, heat the vegetable oil. Add the red onion and cook for about 5 minutes, stirring frequently, until it begins to soften and brown.

3. Add the seitan, cumin, turmeric, paprika, salt, and pepper. Cook, stirring frequently, for about 10 minutes until the seitan browns and some of the edges get crispy.

4. To assemble the sandwiches, stuff each pita with some of the seitan mixture. Add tomato and cucumber slices and romaine lettuce. Drizzle each with the tahini dressing.

5. Substitution tip: Swap store-bought vegan beef for the seitan, if you prefer. You can also use sliced portobello mushrooms to keep your shawarma veggie-centric.

Nutrition:

Calories: 354;

Fat: 12g;

Carbohydrates: 41g;

Fiber: 5g;

Protein: 20g;

Sodium: 718mg;

Chipotle Seitan Taquitos

Preparation time: 15 minutes

Cooking time: 15 minutes

Servings: 12

Ingredients:

- ½ cup Cashew Cream Cheese, or store-bought nondairy cream cheese

- 2 canned chipotle peppers in adobo sauce, minced, sauce reserved

- 12 (6-inch) corn tortillas

- 1 pound Seitan, or store-bought seitan, cut into slices

Directions:

1. Preheat the oven to 400 degreeF. Have a large baking dish or sheet nearby.

2. In a small bowl, stir together the cashew cream cheese, chipotle peppers, and 2 tablespoons of the reserved adobo sauce.

3. Place a tortilla on a clean surface and spread a line (about 2 teaspoons) of the chipotle cream cheese mixture down the middle. Top with a few slices of seitan. Roll up the tortilla as tightly as possible and

place it, seam-side down, in the baking dish. Repeat with the remaining tortillas.

4. Bake for 15 minutes, or until the tortillas are crisp.

Fun fact: Chipotles are not their own type of pepper. They're actually dried, smoked jalapeños. When buying them for this recipe, look for chipotles in adobo sauce, which come in small cans found in the Mexican food section of the grocery store. You'll need both the peppers and the sauce.

Nutrition:

Calories: 193;

Fat: 7g;

Carbohydrates: 25g;

Fiber: 6g;

Protein: 8g;

Sodium: 273mg;

Mediterranean Chickpea Wraps

Preparation time: 15 minutes

Cooking time: 0 minutes

Servings: 4

Ingredients:

- 1/4 cup extra-virgin olive oil

- 2 tablespoons freshly squeezed lemon juice

- 1 teaspoon dried dill

- 1 teaspoon dried oregano

- 1/4 teaspoon salt

- 1 (15-ounce) can chickpeas, drained and rinsed, or 1½ cups cooked chickpeas (see here)

- ½ cup Tofu Feta, or store-bought nondairy feta

- 1 cup chopped cucumber

- 1 large tomato, diced

- ¼ cup diced red onion

- 2 cups fresh baby spinach

- 4 (12-inch) tortillas, or flatbreads of choice

Directions:

1. In a small bowl, whisk the olive oil, lemon juice, dill, oregano, and salt to combine.

2. In a large bowl, gently toss together the chickpeas, feta, cucumber, tomato, and red onion. Add the dressing and toss to combine.

3. Assemble the wraps by placing ½ cup of spinach on each tortilla and topping it with ¼ of the chickpea mixture. Roll up the wrap, tucking in the sides as you go.

Substitution tip: If you'd like to keep your wraps gluten-free and you can't find gluten-free flatbread, use collard greens. You'll need 4 large collard leaves. Cut off the stem from each and shave off the thick part of the stem that's left in the center with a sharp knife. Assemble the wrap the way you would a tortilla, by filling it with the spinach and chickpea mixture and rolling the leaf, tucking in the sides as you go.

Nutrition:

Calories: 623;

Fat: 25g;

Carbohydrates: 80g;

Fiber: 11g;

Protein: 20g;

Sodium: 814mg;

Barbecue Chickpea Burgers With Slaw

Preparation time: 15 minutes

Cooking time: 25 minutes

Servings: 4

Ingredients:

- 1 cup rolled oats

- 1 (15-ounce) can chickpeas, drained and rinsed, or 1½ cup cooked chickpeas (see here)

- ½ cup Barbecue Sauce, or store-bought vegan barbecue sauce, divided

- 1 garlic clove, minced

- ½ teaspoon salt

- ½ teaspoon freshly ground black pepper

- 2 cups shredded cabbage

- 2 carrots, grated or shredded

- ¼ cup Cashew Mayonnaise, or store-bought nondairy mayonnaise

- 4 burger buns of choice

Directions:

1. Preheat the oven to 400 degree F. Line a large baking sheet with parchment paper.

2. In a food processor, pulse the rolled oats until they resemble a coarse meal. Add the chickpeas, ¼ cup of barbecue sauce, the garlic, salt, and pepper.

3. Pulse until the chickpeas are mashed and everything is well combined. It's okay if there are a few whole chickpeas. Form the mixture into 4 patties and place them on the prepared baking sheet.

4. Bake the burgers for 20 to 25 minutes, flipping them at the halfway point. They should be golden brown and firm.

5. While the burgers bake, make the slaw. In a large bowl, stir together the cabbage, carrots, and mayonnaise.

6. Serve each burger on a bun topped with 1 tablespoon of the remaining barbecue sauce and 1/4 cup of slaw.

First-Timer tip: If you don't have a food processor, mash your chickpeas really well using a potato masher or large fork. Rolled oats won't mash well by hand, so use oat flour or all-purpose flour instead. Combine the mashed chickpeas, flour, barbecue sauce, garlic, salt, and pepper in a large bowl before shaping into patties.

Per **serving:**

Calories: 433;

Fat: 10g;

Carbohydrates: 73g;

Fiber: 10g;

Protein: 13g;

Sodium: 665mg;

Sandwiches

Basic Hummus and Vegetable Sandwich

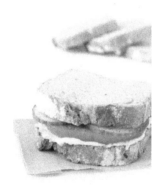

Preparation time: 5 Minutes

Cooking time: 0 Minutes

Servings: 1

Ingredients:

- Salad Greens (1/2 C.)

- Avocado (1/4, Mashed)

- Bell Pepper (1/4, Sliced)

- Hummus (3 T.)

- Whole-grain Bread (2 Slices)

- Carrots (1/4 C., Sliced)

- Cucumber (1/4 C., Sliced)

Directions:

1. For a quick and easy lunch, you will first want to lay the bread out and spread hummus on one side and avocado on the other.

2. Once the spread is placed, put the vegetables in between, and your sandwich is ready to go!

Nutrition:

Calories: 350

Carbs: 45g

Fats: 15g

Proteins: 15g

Green Pesto Sandwich

Preparation time: 5 Minutes

Cooking time: 5 Minutes

Servings: 1

Ingredients:

- Whole Wheat Bread (2 Sliced)

- Vegan Pesto (1 T.)

- Artichoke Hearts (

- Cannellini Beans (1/2 C.)

- Avocado (1/2, Sliced)

- Arugula (1/2 C.)

- Olive Oil (2 T.)

- Pepper (to Taste)

Directions:

1. The first step of making this sandwich will be placing the cannellini beans into a bowl and mashing them with a fork.

2. Once this is done, you can mix in your pesto and spread the mixture on both slices of bread.

3. Next, you are going to place the spinach, avocado, and artichoke hearts in the center and then close your sandwich.

4. With the sandwich set, take a skillet and place it over medium heat. Once warm, toss in some olive oil and grill your sandwich until browned on both sides.

5. Typically, this will only take you about five minutes, and then you can slice and enjoy your sandwich.

Nutrition:

Calories: 350

Carbs: 50g

Fats: 20g

Proteins: 10g

Chickpea Salad Sandwich

Preparation time: 10 Minutes

Cooking time: 0 Minutes

Servings: 4

Ingredients:

- Chickpeas (1 Can)

- Sweet Pickle Relish (2 T.)

- Red Bell Pepper (1/4 C.)

- Celery (1, Chopped)

- Vegan Mayo (1/4 C.)

- Lettuce Leaves (

- Bread (4 Slices)

- Salt (to taste)

- Dill (1/4 t.)

- Onion (2 T., Chopped)

Directions:

1. This sandwich is the vegan version of a tuna sandwich! You can begin the recipe by taking out a mixing bowl and adding in the chickpeas.

2. At this point, mash the chickpeas down and then add in the mayo, dill, relish, celery, onion, and bell pepper.

3. Once you stir everything together, season with salt and pepper to your desired flavoring.

4. Now, lay out your bread and spread one side with the mayo before placing the lettuce and chickpea mixture. Close the sandwich, slice in half, and lunch is served!

Nutrition:

Calories: 200

Carbs: 40g

Fats: 5g

Proteins: 8g

Avocado and White Bean Sandwich

Preparation time: 10 Minutes

Cooking time: 0 Minutes

Servings: 4

Ingredients:

- Whole-grain Bread (8 Sliced)

- Lettuce (3 Leaves)

- Alfalfa Sprouts (1 C.)

- Avocado (1, Sliced)

- Lemon (

- White Beans (1 Can)

- Pepper (to Taste)

Directions:

1. Start this sandwich by first taking your beans and place them into a food processor or blender. You will want to puree the beans until the mixture is smooth.

2. At this point, you can season with pepper, salt, and squeeze the lemon juice in.

3. Now that your bean mix is made go ahead and spread it in between the bread slices. With that in

place, build your sandwich with avocado slices, lettuce, and some alfalfa sprouts.

4. Slice the sandwich, and then you can enjoy it!

Nutrition:

Calories: 300

Carbs: 50g

Fats: 10g

Proteins: 10g

Sweet Potato and Kale Sandwich

Preparation time: 10 Minutes

Cooking time: 30 Minutes

Servings: 4

Ingredients:

- Hummus (1/2 C.)

- Kale (2 C.)

- Salt (to Taste)

- Whole-grain Roll (

- Olive Oil (2 T.)

- Sweet Potato (1, Sliced)

Directions:

1. While this sandwich seems simple, the sweet potato adds nice flavor and texture to switch up your typical sandwich choices. You will want to begin by Preparing the oven to 400.

2. As the oven warms, take out a small mixing bowl and toss your sweet potato pieces in the olive oil, pepper, and salt.

3. When the potato is well coated, lay the pieces across a roasting sheet and pop into the cooker for thirty minutes.

4. At the end of thirty minutes, take out the rolls, and spread hummus on either side. Finally, layer your kale, and sweet potato in between the bread and the sandwich will be all set.

Nutrition:

Calories: 100

Carbs: 10g

Fats: 5g

Proteins: 3g

Wrap

Hummus and Quinoa Wrap

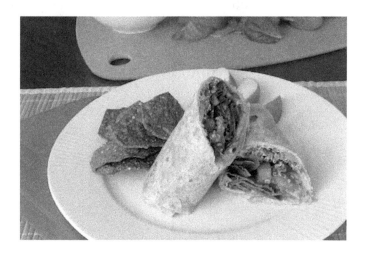

Preparation time: 10 Minutes

Cooking time: 10 Minutes

Servings: 4

Ingredients:

- Lettuce Leaves (

- Cooked Quinoa (1 C.)

- Cabbage (1/2 C.)

- Sprouts (1/2 C.)

- Avocado (1 C., Sliced)

- Hummus (1 C.)

Directions:

1. For this recipe, the lettuce leaves are going to act as your wrap! When you are all set, spread the wrap out and then place the hummus and avocado into each leaf.

2. Once this is set, layer your quinoa and cabbage on top before wrapping the leaf up and eating!

Nutrition:

Calories: 280

Carbs: 40g

Fats: 10g

Proteins: 10g

Conclusion

In a nutshell, this cookbook offers you a world full of options to diversify your plant-based menu. People on this diet are usually seen struggling to choose between healthy food and flavor but, soon, they run out of the options. The selection of 250 recipes in this book is enough to adorn your dinner table with flavorsome, plant-based meals every day. Give each recipe a good read and try them out in the kitchen. You will experience tempting aromas and binding flavors every day.

The book is conceptualized with the idea of offering you a comprehensive view of a plant-based diet and how it can benefit the body. You may find the shift sudden, especially if you are a die-hard fan of non-vegetarian items. But you need not give up anything that you love. Eat everything in moderation.

The next step is to start experimenting with the different recipes in this book and see which ones are your favorites. Everyone has their favorite food, and you will surely find several of yours in this book. Start with breakfast and work your way through. You will be pleasantly surprised at how tasty a vegan meal really can be.

You will love reading this book, as it helps you to understand how revolutionary a plant-based diet can be. It will help you to make informed decisions as you move toward greater change for the greater good. What are you waiting for? Have you begun your journey on the path of the plant-based diet yet? If you haven't, do it now!

Now you have everything you need to get started making budget-friendly, healthy plant-based recipes. Just follow your basic shopping list and follow your meal plan to get started! It's easy to switch over to a plant-based diet if you have your meals planned out and temptation locked away. Don't forget to clean out your kitchen before starting, and you're sure to meet all your diet and health goals.

You need to plan if you are thinking about dieting. First, you can start slowly by just eating one meal a day, which is vegetarian and gradually increasing your number of vegetarian meals. Whenever you are struggling, ask your friend or family member to support you and keep you motivated. One important thing is also to be regularly accountable for not following the diet.

If dieting seems very important to you and you need to do it right, then it is recommended that you visit a professional such as a nutritionist or dietitian to discuss your dieting plan and optimizing it for the better.

No matter how much you want to lose weight, it is not advised that you decrease your calorie intake to an unhealthy level. Losing weight does not mean that you stop eating. It is done by carefully planning meals.

A plant-based diet is very easy once you get into it. At first, you will start to face a lot of difficulties, but if you start slowly, then you can face all the barriers and achieve your goal.

Swap out one unhealthy food item each week that you know is not helping you and put in its place one of the plant-based ingredients that you like. Then have some fun creating the many different recipes in this book. Find out what recipes you like the most so you can make them often and most of all; have some fun exploring all your recipe options.

Wish you good luck with the plant-based diet!